# Instant Pot Ace Blender Cookbook for Beginners

*200 Delicious Recipes to Gain Energy, Lose Weight & Feel Great*

Brence Scoter

# Table of Contents

# Introduction

Kitchen appliances have come a long way in terms of multi-functionality, portability, and competitive prices.

Nowadays, single-use appliances seem lackluster compared to the newer, beautifully crafted, and high-tech cookers.

They have not only become more affordable but are also more energy-efficient. These multi-function appliances are quickly making one-trick appliances obsolete.

When the Instant Pot was introduced in 2010, the market had already seen a slew of other similar cookers.

But despite this, the Instant brand has prevailed over other competitors and rose to become one of America's most loved multi-cooker even to this day.

It quickly gained a following that is at least 2 million and still counting. Patrons around the world who already tried the Instant pot cooker can attest to its versatility.

That is why when Instant pot released yet another multi-function appliance, the Instant Pot Ace blender, patrons were excited and filled with anticipation.

# Chapter 1: An Overview

The products put out by the Instant brand are the result of the genuine love for healthy home-cooked food and the convenience of cooking with pressure and slow cookers.

It is the brainchild of Robert Wang and sold in Canada and the United States in 2010. Over the years, the brand has produced a range of kitchen appliances from pressure cookers, air fryers, rice cookers, blenders, sous vide, toaster ovens, coffee makers, and multi-cookers.

## What is the Instant Pot Ace Blender?

The Instant Pot Ace Blender is far from your typical blender since it can do much more than just blend food.

This one-of-a-kind blender houses a heating element that allows you to cook food before you blend them to make soups, purees, sauces, and more. It also allows users to create cold beverages and soft-serve ice cream to ready to eat hot soups.

What's unique about the Ace blender is that you can put raw vegetables in and end up with hot velvety soup in a short amount of time. It eliminates the need to cook the ingredients before blending, giving you more time to do other things.

The Instant Pot Ace Blender is an affordable appliance that retails only under $100. Right out of the box, the blender has a good weight of about 5kg to give it more stability while in use.

The pitcher is made from a thick heat resistant tempered glass. Other components are manufactured from FDA-approved materials that have fine quality despite being much cheaper than similar blenders in the market.

It is excellent at making milk alternatives from nuts, soy, oats, and rice. The Ace blender can effortlessly make almond and peanut butter, silky flour, frozen desserts, smoothies, and so much more. But one thing that it outshines other similar blenders is its ability to churn out perfect creamy pureed soup every time.

## How Does It Work?

This blender offers different modes that are referred to as programs and offer up to fifteen settings in total.

The manual blending program has low, medium, and high-speed settings that you can use for your usual blending needs.

The blender will only begin to operate after five seconds and will beep three times before commencing. It will also automatically stop after three minutes of blending to prevent overheating. To continue, press the cancel button then select a blending mode again. Once the blender is done with the program, it will beep for 10 times and show done on the digital display.

The hot blending program allows you to choose from among options such as soup, puree, rice milk, and soymilk. The minimum amount of liquid required is 250 ml, while the maximum content should fill only about 1400 ml.

The puree, rice milk, and soup options further allow users to toggle between two cooking options.

The first option under the puree setting is for soft produce, while the second is intended for harder fruits and vegetables.

The first option of the rice milk setting is for white rice, while the second is for brown or any other type of rice you wish to use.

The soup setting will let you choose between chunky or creamy. If you want intermittently stir the ingredients and disable the blending function, you can choose the first option. Make sure that you chop your ingredients the exact sizes you want them to be because the first option will not do any pulverizing.

The heating element at the bottom will cook the ingredients for about 20 minutes after it has reached the boiling point (212 degrees Fahrenheit). The blender will beep to let you know once done.

The second option under the soup setting is for making creamy and velvety soups. Similar to the first option, the blender will cook the ingredients for 20 minutes but blends the ingredients for another two minutes after the cooking is done to give you that creamy consistency.

The cold blending program will let you crush ice, make smoothies, nut milk, and oat milk, as well as, soft-serve ice cream and frozen yogurt. The minimum amount of liquid is 250ml, while the maximum capacity is 1600ml. When using the cold blending program, you must follow this order when adding ingredients to the blender to get the best results.

1. Liquids
2. Powder / sweeteners
3. Leafy greens
4. Soft ingredients
5. Fresh fruits and nuts
6. Frozen fruit
7. Ice cubes

As a safety feature, the blender will not start if the lid is not securely placed. The pause button is helpful when gradually adding ingredients while on a program or if you want to break the cooking cycle for any reason. Simply press the cancel button again, and the cycle will resume. If you want to change the temperature from Celsius to Fahrenheit, press the cancel button once then press and hold the pause button.

The cancel button lets you safely stop the cooking cycle anytime. The Ace blender also features a pulse/clean setting that makes cleaning and maintenance much easier. This setting has 4 cycles lasting for 10 seconds each with 4-second pauses in between to make sure that all remaining dirt and debris are lifted.

## Guide on Care and Maintenance

It is important to clean your blender before using it for the first time and after each subsequent use. Follow these easy steps to properly clean and maintain your cooking blender and keep it in superb working conditions.

### How to use the pulse/clean setting

1. Fill it with 1 liter of hot water and securely cover with the lid.
2. Choose the Pulse/Clean option to shake off and remove any food left on the pitcher.
3. Once the cleaning cycle has ended, discard the contents.
4. Fill the pitcher again with 1 liter of hot water but this time, put some dish soap and repeat steps 2 and 3.
5. Finally, rinse with clear running water before drying and storing.

### Cleaning other parts and components

All removable components such as the lid, lid cap, measuring cup, strainer bag, and food tamper can be hand washed or cleaned with a dishwasher. You may place these items on the top rack when using the dishwasher.

- Always unplug the blender after use and before attempting to take the components out for cleaning.

- Wipe the blender base with a clean damp cloth. Make sure that the unit is unplugged and has cooled down before doing this.
- Wash the strainer bag separately by turning it inside out the letting it completely air dry.
- Do not forget to clean and detach the black silicone from the lid since food can be stuck in these areas too.

Occasional deep cleaning

Deep cleaning your unit from time to time will work wonders in terms of performance. Over time, stains and hard water may build up inside the pitcher. Follow this 3-step process to deep clean your blender whenever necessary.

1. Combine 1 cup each of white vinegar and warm water into the pitcher. Soak for at least 1 hour or longer depending on how tough the stains are.
2. Select the pulse/clean option. Once the cycle is done, unplug the blender and discard the liquid.
3. Rinse with clean running water before drying and storing.

Important maintenance tips

- You may use the cleaning brush that comes with the blender after the cycle is done to make sure that you get all food that may be stuck in the blades.
- Do not leave food inside the pitcher for long periods since this can make clean-up harder.
- Never let the bottom of the pitcher get wet or soaked.
- Make sure to check if the bottom of the pitcher is dry before putting it in the blender base.
- To remove unwanted odors from the silicone lid, simply soak them in equal parts of

water and white vinegar for a couple of hours before rinsing with running water.

- Do not place the blender anywhere near a heat source like burners, ovens, and such as this may damage the unit.
- When storing the blender, never fold the wires tightly to avoid any damage.

## Tips for Successful and Convenient Food Preparation

The excitement of unboxing a new appliance is one of the things that still excite many people. Surely, you are left overwhelmed with all the settings that come with your new cooking blender.

Don't worry you are not alone. Although it comes with a start-up guide and manual, here are more tips you can use to guarantee a stress-free and enjoyable experience when using the Instant Pot Ace Blender.

1. One of the best things you can do after getting your Ace blender is to purchase a cookbook to guide you with recipes that you can try with your new cooking blender. Since the technology is relatively new to a majority of consumers, guides and recipe books are great for maximizing the many functions that your blender has to offer. America's test kitchen offers a comprehensive selection of recipes to get you started on making a variety of meals, drinks, sauces, dips, and desserts with your Instant Pot Ace blender.

2. You may also download the Instant Pot App that is available for mobile users to get access to a bunch of easy to follow recipes you can try with your Ace blender.

3. Never overload the pitcher beyond its recommended amount of contents, as this may cause the motor to overheat.

4. Use the intended settings for the type of foods you are trying to cook or blend. Do not use the hot blending program when making milk from oats, seeds, and nuts.

5. Peel and remove hard shells and seeds from fruits before blending. Tougher produce should be chopped into 1-inch pieces to make blending easier.

6. When making soup with tough vegetables, use the manual blending settings to break them into smaller pieces for it to cook thoroughly.

7. If you want creamier milk from your nuts or seeds, simply soak them overnight before blending. You can add salt, cocoa powder, vanilla, or cinnamon to your milk to add extra flavor.

8. Carbonated liquids are not suitable for use in the Ace blender as it produces a lot of foam that may overflow and go beyond the blender's capacity.

9. You can quickly use a microwave to brown or soften tough ingredients before adding into the blender to add added flavors to your soups.

10. When using the hot blending program, keep oven mitts or tea towels nearby. The pitcher and cover can get hot and you will need these if you have to add any ingredients while cooking.

11. Keep your blender blades sharp by using at least 4 dry eggshells and 1-2 cups of water. Run your blender in the pulse mode, pour out the contents, then rinse.

# Chapter 2: Beverages & Smoothies

## Orange, Banana & Strawberry Smoothie

Preparation Time: 5 minutes

Cooking Time: 0 minute

Servings: 4

Ingredients:

- 2 cups orange juice
- 2 bananas, sliced
- 2 1/2 cups strawberries, sliced
- 1 tablespoon honey
- 1 1/2 cups ice

Method:

1. Pour orange juice into the Instant Pot Ace Blender.
2. Add bananas and strawberries.
3. Drizzle honey on top.
4. Top with ice.
5. Secure the blender with the lid.
6. Set it to smoothie program.
7. Set it to 1:38 minutes.

Serving Suggestions: Garnish with strawberry slices.

Preparation & Cooking Tips: To make your smoothie creamier, you can add vanilla yogurt into the mix. You can also make it dairy free by using soy milk.

# Frozen Mochaccinos

Preparation Time: 5 minutes

Cooking Time: 0 minute

Servings: 4

Ingredients:

- 2 cups milk
- 1/4 teaspoon vanilla extract
- 1/4 cup chocolate syrup
- 1 tablespoon coffee
- 2 tablespoons sugar
- 3 cups ice

Method:

1. Combine all ingredients except whipped cream in the Instant Pot Ace Blender.
2. Lock the lid in place.
3. Press the smoothie program.
4. Set it to 1:38 minutes.

Serving Suggestions: Garnish with whipped cream.

Preparation & Cooking Tips: You can replace sugar with agave nectar if you like.

# Angel Food Smoothie

Preparation Time: 5 minutes

Cooking Time: 0 minute

Servings: 2

Ingredients:

- 1/4 cup water
- 1 banana, sliced
- 3/4 cup strawberries, sliced
- 2 tablespoons sugar
- 2 tablespoons milk
- 2 drops vanilla extract
- 1 1/2 cups ice

Method:

1. Pour water into the Instant Pot Ace Blender.
2. Stir in banana and strawberries.
3. Add sugar, milk and vanilla.
4. Top with ice.
5. Secure lid in place.
6. Select smoothie program.
7. Press start button.
8. Pulse until smooth.

Serving Suggestions: Garnish with strawberry slices.

Preparation & Cooking Tips: Use ripe bananas for this recipe.

# Peach Cobbler Smoothie

Preparation Time: 5 minutes

Cooking Time: 0 minute

Servings: 2

Ingredients:

- 1/2 cup milk
- 1 tablespoon honey
- 1/2 cup plain yogurt
- 1/8 teaspoon ground ginger
- 1/8 teaspoon nutmeg
- 1/8 teaspoon cinnamon powder
- 1 cup peaches, sliced

Method:

1. In a bowl, mix milk, honey, yogurt, ground ginger, nutmeg and cinnamon powder.
2. Pour mixture into the Instant Pot Ace Blender.
3. Stir in peaches.
4. Press smoothie program.
5. Process until smooth.

Serving Suggestions: Top with chopped peaches.

Preparation & Cooking Tips: You can also use vanilla extract in place of honey.

# Horchata

Preparation Time: 35 minutes

Cooking Time: 15 minutes

Servings: 4

Ingredients:

- 1/2 cup white rice
- 1 teaspoon vegetable oil
- 4 cups water
- 1/3 cup granulated sugar
- 1/4 teaspoon ground cinnamon

Method:

1. Add rice, oil and water to the Instant Pot Ace Blender.
2. Choose rice milk 1 setting.
3. Carefully uncover the blender.
4. Pour mixture to a strainer bag.
5. Put the strained rice milk back to the blender.
6. Add the rest of the ingredients.
7. Choose low manual setting.
8. Set it to 10 seconds.
9. Chill in the refrigerator for 30 minutes and serve.

Serving Suggestions: Sprinkle with ground cinnamon on top before serving.

Preparation & Cooking Tips: You can add more water when you blend the ingredients to thin the consistency.

# Green Smoothie

Preparation Time: 5 minutes

Cooking Time: 0 minute

Servings: 2

Ingredients:

- 4 dates, pitted
- 3 cups baby spinach
- 2 bananas, sliced
- 2 tablespoon almonds
- 1 tablespoon peanut butter
- 1 cup ice cubes

Method:

1. Mix all ingredients in the Instant Pot Ace Blender.
2. Seal the blender.
3. Press smoothie setting.
4. Pulse until smooth.

Serving Suggestions: Garnish with chia seeds or flaxseeds.

Preparation & Cooking Tips: Use natural peanut butter for this recipe.

# Peanut Butter Smoothie with Banana

Preparation Time: 5 minutes

Cooking Time: 0 minute

Servings: 2

Ingredients:

- 1 cup almond milk
- 1/4 cup quick oats
- 3 dates, pitted
- 2 bananas, sliced
- 1/3 cup peanut butter
- 1/2 cup ice

Method:

1. Pour almond milk into the Instant Pot Ace Blender.
2. Stir in oats, dates, bananas and peanut butter.
3. Top with ice.
4. Seal the blender.
5. Press smoothie setting.
6. Press pulse and then start.
7. Pulse three times.
8. Press cancel to stop blending.

Serving Suggestions: Top with a dollop of peanut butter.

Preparation & Cooking Tips: It's also a good idea to freeze banana slices first before blending.

# Super Smoothie

Preparation Time: 5 minutes

Cooking Time: 2 minutes

Servings: 4

Ingredients:

- 2 1/4 cups soy milk
- 1 cup kale, chopped
- 1 cup baby spinach, chopped
- 2 tablespoon agave nectar
- 1 1/2 cups mango, sliced
- 1 1/2 cups peaches, sliced

Method:

1. Pour soy milk into the Instant Pot Ace Blender.
2. Add kale, spinach, agave nectar, mango and peaches to the blender.
3. Seal the blender with its lid.
4. Select smoothie program.
5. Set it to 1:38 minutes.

Serving Suggestions: Garnish with mango or peach slices.

Preparation & Cooking Tips: You can also use almond milk instead of soy milk.

# Strawberry Milkshake

Preparation Time: 5 minutes

Cooking Time: 0 minute

Servings: 4

Ingredients:

- 2 cups milk
- 4 cups strawberries, sliced
- 3 tablespoons vanilla extract

Method:

1. Combine milk, strawberries and vanilla extract in the Instant Pot Ace Blender.
2. Lock the lid in place.
3. Press smoothie setting.
4. Set it to 1:38 minutes.

Serving Suggestions: Top with chopped strawberries.

Preparation & Cooking Tips: If you want your milkshake dairy free, use almond milk instead of cow's milk.

# Creamy Banana & Strawberry Smoothie

Preparation Time: 5 minutes

Cooking Time: 0 minute

Servings: 2

Ingredients:

- 1 cup almond milk
- 1 cup strawberries, chopped
- 2 cups banana slices
- 1/2 cup vanilla yogurt

Method:

1. Add all ingredients to the Instant Pot Ace Blender.
2. Seal the blender.
3. Choose smoothie program.
4. Pulse until smooth.

Serving Suggestions: Drizzle with almond milk on top.

Preparation & Cooking Tips: You can add honey to sweeten your smoothie.

# Pineapple & Mango Smoothie

Preparation Time: 5 minutes

Cooking Time: 0 minute

Servings: 2

Ingredients:

- 1 cup almond milk
- 2 cups mango, slices
- 2 cups pineapple chunks
- 1 cup ice

Method:

1. Pour almond milk into the Instant Pot Ace Blender.
2. Add mango and pineapple chunks.
3. Top with ice.
4. Lock the lid in place.
5. Choose smoothie program.
6. Set it to 1:38 minutes.

Serving Suggestions: Garnish with pineapple slice.

Preparation & Cooking Tips: You can add more tropical fruits to this recipe if you like.

# Loaded Berry Smoothie

Preparation Time: 5 minutes

Cooking Time: 0 minute

Servings: 4

Ingredients:

- 1 teaspoon lemon juice
- 2 cups strawberries, chopped
- 1 cup blueberries, sliced in half
- 1 cup raspberries, sliced in half
- 2 tablespoons honey
- 1/2 cup ice cubes

Method:

1. Pour lemon juice into the Instant Pot Ace Blender.
2. Add the berries to the blender.
3. Drizzle with honey.
4. Top with ice.
5. Seal the blender.
6. Press smoothie program.
7. Pulse until berries are fully combined.

Serving Suggestions: Garnish with berries.

Preparation & Cooking Tips: You can also add blackberries to the mix if you like.

# Cucumber & Lemon Smoothie

Preparation Time: 5 minutes

Cooking Time: 0 minute

Servings: 2

Ingredients:

- 2 cups cucumber, sliced
- 1 cup lemon juice
- 2 tablespoons honey
- 1 cup ice

Method:

1. Add all ingredients to the Instant Pot Ace Blender.
2. Secure the lid of the blender.
3. Press smoothie setting.
4. Set it to 1:40 minutes.

Serving Suggestions: Garnish with lemon wedges.

Preparation & Cooking Tips: You can freeze cucumber before blending.

# Sunrise Smoothie

Preparation Time: 5 minutes

Cooking Time: 0 minute

Servings: 2

Ingredients:

- 1 banana, sliced
- 1 apricot, sliced
- 1 cup peach yogurt
- 1 tablespoon lemonade concentrate
- 1 cup club soda
- 1 cup ice

Method:

1. Combine banana, apricot, yogurt, lemonade concentrate, club soda and ice in the Instant Pot Ace Blender.
2. Cover the blender.
3. Press smoothie program.
4. Set it to 1:40 minutes.

Serving Suggestions: Top with chopped peaches.

Preparation & Cooking Tips: Use low-fat peach yogurt.

# Berry & Vanilla Smoothie

Preparation Time: 5 minutes

Cooking Time: 0 minute

Servings: 2

Ingredients:

- 1 cup raspberries, sliced in half
- 1 cup strawberries, sliced in half
- 1 cup pineapple juice (unsweetened)
- 1 cup vanilla yogurt
- 1/2 cup ice

Method:

1. Add fruits, juice and yogurt to the Instant Pot Ace Blender.
2. Lock the lid in place.
3. Select smoothie program.
4. Set it to 1:40 minutes.

Serving Suggestions: Garnish with berries.

Preparation & Cooking Tips: Use fat-free vanilla yogurt.

# Citrusy Berry Shake

Preparation Time: 5 minutes

Cooking Time: 0 minute

Servings: 2

Ingredients:

- 1 cup orange juice
- 1 tablespoon pineapple juice
- 1/2 cup strawberries, sliced
- 1/2 cup blueberries, sliced
- 1/2 cup blackberries, sliced
- 1/2 cup pineapple chunks
- 1/2 cup banana, sliced
- 1/2 cup plain Greek yogurt

Method:

1. Stir all ingredients to the Instant Pot Ace Blender.
2. Seal the blender.
3. Choose smoothie setting.
4. Process for 2 minutes.

Serving Suggestions: Top with chopped mixed berries.

Preparation & Cooking Tips: You can also use frozen mixed berry for this recipe.

# Strawberry Smoothie with Pumpkin Seeds

Preparation Time: 5 minutes

Cooking Time: 0 minute

Servings: 1

Ingredients:

- 1 cup skim milk
- 1 cup frozen strawberries, sliced
- 1 tablespoon flaxseed oil
- 1 tablespoon pumpkin seeds

Method:

1. Add all the ingredients to the Instant Pot Ace Blender.
2. Seal the blender.
3. Select smoothie setting.
4. Process for 2 minutes or until smooth.

Serving Suggestions: Top with pumpkin seeds.

Preparation & Cooking Tips: You can also use sunflower seeds for this recipe.

# Creamy Blueberry Smoothie

Preparation Time: 5 minutes

Cooking Time: 0 minute

Servings: 2

Ingredients:

- 1 cup frozen blueberries
- 1/2 cup yogurt
- 1 cup orange juice

Method:

1. Add berries, yogurt and orange juice to the Instant Pot Ace Blender.
2. Cover the blender.
3. Set it to smoothie.
4. Set time to 30 seconds.
5. Process and serve in glasses.

Serving Suggestions: Garnish with chopped blueberries.

Preparation & Cooking Tips: Use Greek yogurt for this recipe.

# Banana Soy Smoothie

Preparation Time: 5 minutes

Cooking Time: 0 minute

Servings: 1

Ingredients:

- 1 cup soy milk
- 1/2 cup blueberries
- 1 banana, sliced
- 1 cup ice

Method:

1. Pour soy milk into the Instant Pot Ace Blender.
2. Add blueberries and banana.
3. Top with ice.
4. Lock the lid in place.
5. Select smoothie function.
6. Set it to 1 minute.
7. Process and serve.

Serving Suggestions: Top with cereal flakes.

Preparation & Cooking Tips: You can replace blueberries with blackberries or raspberries.

# Mango, Banana & Pineapple Smoothie

Preparation Time: 5 minutes

Cooking Time: 0 minute

Servings: 2

Ingredients:

- 1 cup vanilla yogurt
- 2 cups pineapple chunks
- 1 banana, sliced
- 1 mango, sliced into cubes
- 2 cup ice cubes

Method:

1. Add yogurt to the Instant Pot Ace Blender.
2. Stir in pineapple, banana and mango.
3. Seal the blender.
4. Process until smooth.
5. Add ice.
6. Blend until fully combined.

Serving Suggestions: Top with a dollop of yogurt.

Preparation & Cooking Tips: Freeze yogurt before blending.

# Banana & Ginger

Preparation Time: 5 minutes

Cooking Time: 0 minute

Servings: 2

Ingredients:

- 2 bananas, sliced
- 1 cup vanilla yogurt
- 1/2 teaspoon ground ginger
- 2 tablespoons honey

Method:

1. Place all the ingredients in the Instant Pot Ace Blender.
2. Secure the lid.
3. Select smoothie function.
4. Set it to 1:38 minutes.
5. Process and serve.

Serving Suggestions: Top with a dollop of yogurt.

Preparation & Cooking Tips: You can also use minced fresh ginger for this recipe.

# Creamy Orange Shake

Preparation Time: 5 minutes

Cooking Time: 0 minute

Servings: 2

Ingredients:

- 1/4 cup half and half
- 2 tablespoons orange juice concentrate
- 1/2 teaspoon vanilla extra
- 2 cups ice

Method:

1. Pour half and half, orange juice concentrate and vanilla extract to the Instant Pot Ace Blender.
2. Mix with a ladle.
3. Add the ice on top.
4. Secure the lid.
5. Press smoothie program.
6. Process until smooth.

Serving Suggestions: Garnish with orange slice.

Preparation & Cooking Tips: Use nonfat half and half to lower calorie and fat content of this recipe.

# Green Tea Smoothie with Banana & Blueberry

Preparation Time: 5 minutes

Cooking Time: 5 minutes

Servings: 2

Ingredients:

- 1 cup green tea leaves
- 2 cups banana, sliced
- 2 cups blueberry, sliced
- 1 cup vanilla soy milk
- 1 cup ice

Method:

1. Add green tea leaves to a pot over medium heat.
2. Boil for 5 minutes.
3. Strain the mixture.
4. Let tea cool in a cup.
5. Pour tea into the Instant Pot Ace Blender.
6. Stir in the rest of the ingredients.
7. Secure the lid.
8. Choose smoothie program.
9. Blend until smooth.

Serving Suggestions: Garnish with banana or blueberry slice.

Preparation & Cooking Tips: You can also use green tea bag for this recipe and steep in hot water for 5 minutes.

# Cherry & Berry Smoothie

Preparation Time: 5 minutes

Cooking Time: 0 minute

Servings: 2

Ingredients:

- 1 cup almond milk
- 1 cup raspberries
- 1/4 cup cherries, pitted and sliced
- 2 teaspoons ginger, grated
- 1 teaspoon ground flaxseed
- 2 teaspoons lemon juice

Method:

1. Pour almond milk into the Instant Pot Ace Blender.
2. Add the rest of the ingredients.
3. Mix with a spoon.
4. Lock the lid in place.
5. Choose smoothie program.
6. Set it to 2 minutes.
7. Process and serve.

Serving Suggestions: Garnish with a cherry.

Preparation & Cooking Tips: You can also use minced fresh ginger.

# Kiwi Strawberry Smoothie

Preparation Time: 5 minutes

Cooking Time: 0 minute

Servings: 2

Ingredients:

- 2 cups apple juice
- 1 kiwi, sliced
- 1 cup strawberries, sliced
- 1 banana, sliced
- 2 teaspoons honey
- 1 cup ice

Method:

1. Pour apple juice into the Instant Pot Ace Blender.
2. Stir in kiwi, strawberries and banana.
3. Drizzle with honey.
4. Top with ice.
5. Lock the lid in place.
6. Select smoothie function.
7. Set time to 1:38 minutes.
8. Process and serve.

Serving Suggestions: Garnish with kiwi slice.

Preparation & Cooking Tips: You can also use agave nectar for this recipe.

# Blueberry & Soy Smoothie

Preparation Time: 5 minutes

Cooking Time: 0 minute

Servings: 2

Ingredients:

- 2 cups soy milk
- 1 banana, sliced
- 1 cup blueberries
- 1/4 cup milk
- 1 teaspoon vanilla extract
- 1 cup ice

Method:

1. Pour soy milk to the Instant Pot Ace Blender.
2. Add banana and blueberries.
3. Stir milk and vanilla extract.
4. Top with ice.
5. Seal the blender.
6. Choose smoothie function.
7. Set it to 1:38 minutes.
8. Process and serve.

Serving Suggestions: Drizzle with milk on top before serving.

Preparation & Cooking Tips: You can also use almond milk if you don't have soy milk.

# Coconut & Papaya Shake

Preparation Time: 5 minutes

Cooking Time: 0 minute

Servings: 2

Ingredients:

- 1 cup pineapple chunks
- 2 cups papaya, sliced
- 1 cup plain yogurt
- 1 tablespoons coconut flake
- 1 teaspoon ground flaxseed
- 1 cup ice

Method:

1. Combine all ingredients in the Instant Pot Ace Blender.
2. Seal the blender.
3. Press smoothie function.
4. Press start to pulse for 30 seconds to 1 minute or until smooth.
5. Press cancel to stop blending.

Serving Suggestions: Top with coconut flakes.

Preparation & Cooking Tips: Use low-fat Greek yogurt.

# Peach & Strawberry Smoothie

Preparation Time: 5 minutes

Cooking Time: 0 minute

Servings: 2

Ingredients:

- 2 tablespoons vanilla yogurt
- 1 cup milk
- 2 teaspoon protein powder
- Pinch ground ginger
- 1/2 cup peaches
- 1/2 cup strawberries
- 1 cup ice cubes

Method:

1. Add vanilla yogurt, milk, protein powder and ginger to the Instant Pot Ace Blender.
2. Select smoothie function.
3. Press start to pulse for 30 seconds.
4. Press cancels.
5. Stir in the remaining ingredients.
6. Set it to 1:38 minutes.
7. Process and serve.

Serving Suggestions: Top with chopped strawberries.

Preparation & Cooking Tips: You can use almond or soy milk to make this recipe dairy free.

# Lemon, Mango & Yogurt Smoothie

Preparation Time: 5 minutes

Cooking Time: 0 minute

Servings: 2

Ingredients:

- 2 mangoes, sliced
- 1 cup milk
- 1/2 cup yogurt
- 2 tablespoons lemon juice
- 1 teaspoon vanilla extract
- 1 teaspoon lemon zest
- 1 cup ice cubes

Method:

1. Put all the ingredients in the Instant Pot Ace Blender, adding the ice last.
2. Seal the blender.
3. Press smoothie function.
4. Set it to 1:38 minutes.
5. Process and serve.

Serving Suggestions: Sprinkle lemon zest on top.

Preparation & Cooking Tips: Use freshly squeezed lemon juice.

# Watermelon Smoothie

Preparation Time: 5 minutes

Cooking Time: 0 minute

Servings: 2

Ingredients:

- 2 cups watermelon, chopped
- 1/4 cup milk
- 2 cups ice

Method:

1. Mix all ingredients in the Instant Pot Ace Blender.
2. Secure the lid.
3. Choose smoothie function.
4. Pulse for 30 seconds.
5. Press cancels.
6. Serve.

Serving Suggestions: Garnish with watermelon slice.

Preparation & Cooking Tips: It's also a good idea to freeze watermelon slices before blending.

# Chapter 3: Soups

## Chicken Noodle Soup

Preparation Time: 15 minutes

Cooking Time: 20 minutes

Servings: 4

Ingredients:

- 1 tablespoon olive oil
- 4 cups chicken stock
- 1/2 cup yellow onion
- 1/4 cup celery, chopped
- 1 cup carrot, chopped
- 1/4 teaspoon dried rosemary
- 3/4 teaspoon dried thyme
- Salt to taste
- 1 pack rotini pasta
- 1 cup cooked chicken, shredded

Method:

1. Pour olive oil and chicken stock to the Instant Pot Ace Blender.
2. Add onion, celery, carrot, herbs and salt.
3. Stir.
4. Lock the lid in place.
5. Select soup function.
6. Set it to 20 minutes.

7. Press pause when the cooking in the last 2 minutes.

8. Stir in the pasta and chicken.

9. Continue cooking.

10. Transfer to a bowl and serve.

**Serving Suggestions:** Garnish with chopped parsley.

**Preparation & Cooking Tips:** You can also make chicken and rice soup version of this recipe.

# Tomato Soup

Preparation Time: 15 minutes

Cooking Time: 23 minutes

Servings: 4

Ingredients:

- 2 cups vegetable stock
- 28 oz. canned whole tomatoes, liquid undrained
- 1 onion, chopped
- 3 cloves garlic, minced
- 1 1/2 tablespoons sugar
- 3 tablespoons tomato paste
- 1 teaspoon Italian seasoning
- Salt and pepper to taste
- 3 tablespoons butter

Method:

1. Add vegetable stock, tomatoes, onion, garlic, sugar, tomatoes with liquid, Italian seasoning, salt and pepper to the Instant Pot Ace Blender.
2. Seal the blender.
3. Select soup function.
4. Set it to 22:44 minutes.
5. Add butter before serving.

Serving Suggestions: Garnish with fresh basil.

Preparation & Cooking Tips: Stir 1/2 teaspoon baking soda into the soup after cooking to neutralize acidity of tomatoes.

# Chicken & Lime Soup

Preparation Time: 5 minutes
Cooking Time: 25 minutes
Servings: 4

Ingredients:

- 1 onion, chopped
- 2 cloves garlic, minced
- 1 stalk celery, chopped
- 1 tablespoon olive oil
- 1 jalapeno pepper, chopped
- 8 oz. chicken breast, chopped
- 14 oz. diced tomatoes
- 3 cups chicken broth
- 1/2 teaspoon cumin
- 1/2 teaspoon dried oregano
- Salt to taste
- 3 tablespoon cilantro leaves
- 1 tablespoon lime juice

Method:

1. Add onion, garlic, celery, olive oil, jalapeno, chicken, tomatoes, broth, cumin, oregano and salt to the Instant Pot Ace Blender.
2. Choose soup 1 function.
3. Stir in cilantro and lime juice.
4. Press low setting and pulse for 3 seconds.

Serving Suggestions: Garnish with lime wedges.

Preparation & Cooking Tips: Use low-sodium chicken stock.

# Sausage Chili

Preparation Time: 20 minutes

Cooking Time: 20 minutes

Servings: 4

Ingredients:

- 1/2 red onion, diced
- 1/2 yellow bell pepper, diced
- 1 jalapeno pepper, diced
- 10 oz. canned diced tomatoes
- 14 oz. canned diced tomatoes, liquid undrained
- 3 tablespoon tomato paste
- 7 oz. sausage, chopped
- 1 tablespoon chili powder
- 1 teaspoon ground cumin
- 1/4 teaspoon garlic powder
- 3 tablespoons fresh cilantro, chopped
- Salt and pepper to taste
- 15 oz. red kidney beans, drained
- Cheddar cheese, shredded

Method:

1. Combine all the ingredients except kidney beans and cheddar cheese into the Instant Pot Ace Blender.
2. Seal the blender.
3. Select soup program and set it to 20 minutes.

4. Press pause in the last 5 minutes of cooking.

5. Add kidney beans and continue cooking.

6. Top with cheese.

Serving Suggestions: Garnish with sour cream.

Preparation & Cooking Tips: You can also use smoked sausage for this recipe.

# Corn Chowder

Preparation Time: 15 minutes

Cooking Time: 20 minutes

Servings: 4

Ingredients:

- 3 cups chicken stock
- 1/2 onion, diced
- 3 1/2 cups corn kernels
- 1 tablespoon sugar
- 1 teaspoon dried thyme
- 1/4 teaspoon onion powder
- Salt and pepper to taste
- 1 teaspoon cornstarch mixed into 2 tablespoons water
- 1/3 cup red bell pepper, diced
- 1/3 cup heavy cream
- Bacon, cooked crisp and crumbled

Method:

1. Pour chicken stock into the Instant Pot Ace Blender.
2. Add onion, corn, sugar, thyme, onion powder, salt and pepper.
3. Seal the blender.
4. Select soup program.
5. Set it to 20 minutes.
6. Press pause in the last 5 minutes of cooking.
7. Add cornstarch mixture and bell pepper.

8. Continue cooking.

9. Stir in cream and top with bacon bits.

Serving Suggestions: Garnish with fresh herbs.

Preparation & Cooking Tips: You can also use chopped ham in place of bacon.

# Butternut Squash Soup

Preparation Time: 15 minutes

Cooking Time: 25 minutes

Servings: 4

Ingredients:

- 2 1/4 cups chicken stock
- 1/4 onion, chopped
- 1 tablespoon honey
- 24 oz. butternut squash, sliced into cubes
- 1/8 teaspoon ground nutmeg
- 1/4 teaspoon dried thyme
- Salt and pepper to taste
- 2 tablespoon vegetable oil spread
- 3 leaves sage, minced

Method:

1. Pour chicken stock into the Instant Pot Ace Blender.
2. Add the rest of the ingredients except vegetable oil spread and sage.
3. Seal the blender.
4. Select soup function and set it to 22:44 minutes.
5. Add vegetable oil spread and sage.

Serving Suggestions: Garnish with pumpkin seeds.

Preparation & Cooking Tips: You can also use vegetable stock in place of chicken stock, and pumpkin instead of squash.

# Cauliflower Soup

Preparation Time: 5 minutes

Cooking Time: 40 minutes

Servings: 4

Ingredients:

- 30 oz. cauliflower florets
- 2 cups chicken broth
- 1 1/2 teaspoons onion powder
- 1 1/2 teaspoons garlic powder
- 8 oz. cream cheese
- 1 teaspoon Dijon mustard
- 1 teaspoon hot sauce
- Salt and pepper to taste

Method:

1. Put all the ingredients in the Instant Pot Ace Blender.
2. Seal the blender.
3. Press soup 2 setting.
4. Process and serve.

Serving Suggestions: Garnish with chopped parsley.

Preparation & Cooking Tips: You can also stir a tablespoon of parsley into the soup before serving.

# Tomato & Basil Soup

Preparation Time: 5 minutes

Cooking Time: 20 minutes

Servings: 4

Ingredients:

- 28 oz. canned tomatoes
- 1/2 tablespoon dried basil
- 2 oz. cheddar cheese
- 4 tablespoon heavy whipping cream
- Garlic salt to taste

Method:

1. Mix all the ingredients in the Instant Pot Ace Blender.
2. Choose soup 1 setting.
3. Set it to 20 minutes.

Serving Suggestions: Garnish with shredded cheese.

Preparation & Cooking Tips: You can use any type of hard cheese for garnish.

# Carrot Soup with Spices

Preparation Time: 10 minutes

Cooking Time: 50 minutes

Servings: 6

Ingredients:

- 2 lb. carrots, sliced into cubes
- 2 cups water
- 2 tablespoon olive oil
- 2 onions, chopped
- Salt and pepper to taste
- 1 tablespoon ginger, grated
- 1 tablespoon ground fennel
- 1 teaspoon ground cinnamon
- 1 tablespoon ground coriander
- 4 cups vegetable broth

Method:

1. Add carrots and water to the Instant Pot Ace Blender.
2. Select puree setting.
3. Blend carrots until pureed.
4. Transfer to a pot over medium heat.
5. Stir in the rest of the ingredients.
6. Bring to a boil.
7. Simmer for 10 minutes.

Serving Suggestions: Top with cilantro and hazelnuts.

Preparation & Cooking Tips: You can also add plain Greek yogurt to the soup to make it creamy.

# Refried Bean & Vegetable Soup

Preparation Time: 10 minutes

Cooking Time: 20 minutes

Servings: 4

Ingredients:

- 16 oz. beef broth
- 1 teaspoon chili powder
- 1/2 teaspoon tomato powder
- 2 teaspoons taco seasoning
- 1 onion, sliced
- 1 clove garlic, peeled
- 1 red pepper, sliced
- 1 stalk celery, chopped
- 1 carrot, sliced
- 1/4 cup mushrooms, sliced
- 14 oz. refried beans
- 3 teaspoons lemon juice

Method:

1. Pour beef broth to the Instant Pot Ace Blender.
2. Stir in chili powder, tomato powder and taco seasoning.
3. Add onion, garlic, red pepper, celery, carrot, mushrooms and refried beans.
4. Stir in lemon juice.
5. Select soup 1 function and set it to 20 minutes.

Serving Suggestions: Garnish with cilantro.

Preparation & Cooking Tips: Use freshly squeezed lemon juice.

# Potato & Leek Soup

Preparation Time: 20 minutes

Cooking Time: 25 minutes

Servings: 4

Ingredients:

- 3 cups vegetable stock
- 2 potatoes, chopped
- 1 leek, chopped
- 2 cloves garlic
- 3/4 teaspoon dried thyme
- Salt and pepper to taste

Method:

1. Pour vegetable stock into the Instant Pot Ace Blender.
2. Add the rest of the ingredients.
3. Seal the blender.
4. Press soup program and set it to 22:44 minutes.

Serving Suggestions: Top with heavy cream.

Preparation & Cooking Tips: You can also top with crumbled crispy bacon bits.

# Clam Chowder

Preparation Time: 5 minutes

Cooking Time: 40 minutes

Servings: 4

Ingredients:

- 12 oz. canned clams, minced
- 1 onion, chopped
- 1 tablespoon tomato paste
- 30 oz. canned diced tomatoes
- 1/2 teaspoon dried marjoram
- 2 cups potatoes, diced
- 1 cup celery, chopped
- Pepper to taste

Method:

1. Add clam meat with its juice to the Instant Pot Ace Blender.
2. Stir in onion and tomato paste.
3. Seal the blender.
4. Press pulse and start.
5. Pulse until fully combined.
6. Add the rest of the ingredients.
7. Mix.
8. Choose soup program.
9. Set it to 15 minutes.

Serving Suggestions: Sprinkle with crispy bacon bits.

Preparation & Cooking Tips: You can also use fresh clam meat.

# Squash Noodle Soup

Preparation Time: 10 minutes

Cooking Time: 35 minutes

Servings: 4

Ingredients:

- 4 cups chicken broth
- 1 cup bowtie pasta
- 1/4 cup fresh basil, sliced
- 1/2 teaspoon oregano, chopped
- 1/2 teaspoon thyme, chopped
- Pepper to taste
- 2 cups squash, diced
- 1 cup zucchini, diced

Method:

1. Pour broth into the Instant Pot Ace Blender.
2. Seal the blender.
3. Press soup setting.
4. Set it to 15 minutes.
5. After 15 minutes, press pause.
6. Add pasta and set it to 5:30 minutes.
7. After this, add the rest of the ingredients.
8. Mix well.
9. Set it to 15 minutes.

Serving Suggestions: Serve with shaved Parmesan cheese on top.

Preparation & Cooking Tips: Use vegetable stock if you want to turn this recipe into vegetarian.

# Spinach & Tomato Soup

Preparation Time: 15 minutes

Cooking Time: 17 minutes

Servings: 4

Ingredients:

- 3 cups chicken broth
- 15 oz. canned diced tomatoes
- 15 oz. canned kidney beans
- 1 teaspoon Italian seasoning
- 1/2 teaspoon smoked paprika
- Salt and pepper to taste
- 4 cups spinach

Method:

1. Pour broth into the Instant Pot Ace Blender.
2. Add tomatoes, beans and seasonings to the blender.
3. Seal the blender.
4. Press soup setting.
5. Set it to 15:00 minutes.
6. Stir in spinach and let it sit for 2 minutes before serving.

Serving Suggestions: Sprinkle with grated Parmesan cheese on top.

Preparation & Cooking Tips: You can also use arugula for this recipe.

# Corn Soup

Preparation Time: 10 minutes

Cooking Time: 20 minutes

Servings: 4

Ingredients:

- 2 1/4 cups broth
- 1 onion, sliced into wedges
- 1 clove garlic, minced
- 4 cups corn kernels
- 1/2 lb. potatoes, sliced into cubes
- 1 bay leaf
- 2 teaspoons fresh thyme, chopped
- 1/4 cup heavy cream

Method:

1. Pour broth into the Instant Pot Ace Blender.
2. Add onion, garlic, corn kernels and potatoes.
3. Pulse until smooth.
4. Add the thyme and bay leaf.
5. Press soup setting and set it to 10:00 minutes.
6. Stir in cream.
7. Set it to 10:00 minutes more.

Serving Suggestions: Sprinkle with chopped chives on top.

Preparation & Cooking Tips: Stir in a teaspoon of honey to sweeten the soup.

# Chickpea Soup

Preparation Time: 10 minutes

Cooking Time: 25 minutes

Servings: 4

Ingredients:

- 1 1/2 cups vegetable broth
- 1 onion, sliced
- 1 carrot, sliced
- 15 oz. chickpeas, rinsed and drained
- 14 oz. coconut milk
- Salt and pepper to taste

Method:

1. Add all the ingredients to the Instant Pot Ace Blender.
2. Select soup 2 setting.
3. Set it to 15:00 minutes.

Serving Suggestions: Top with minced carrots.

Preparation & Cooking Tips: You can also add curry powder to this recipe.

# Cheesy Cauliflower Soup

Preparation Time: 10 minutes

Cooking Time: 20 minutes

Servings: 4

Ingredients:

- 3 cups vegetable broth
- 4 cups cauliflower florets
- 2 teaspoon vegetable bouillon powder
- Garlic salt to taste
- Cheddar cheese

Method:

1. Add vegetable broth to the Instant Pot Ace Blender.
2. Stir in the rest of the ingredients except the cheese.
3. Press soup setting.
4. Set it to 20:00 minutes.
5. Add cheese before serving.

Serving Suggestions: Top with toasted pine nuts.

Preparation & Cooking Tips: You can also use Parmesan cheese for this recipe.

# Cheesy Pea Soup

Preparation Time: 20 minutes

Cooking Time: 15 minutes

Servings: 6

Ingredients:

- 1 onion, chopped
- 2 cloves garlic, minced
- 3 stalks celery, chopped
- 3 potatoes, sliced and boiled
- 1 carrot, chopped and boiled
- 2 cups green split peas, rinsed, drained and boiled
- 1 teaspoon liquid smoke
- 1 teaspoon dried marjoram
- 1 teaspoon dried basil
- 1 bay leaf
- Salt and pepper to taste
- 1 cup nacho cheese sauce

Method:

1. Add onion, garlic, celery, potatoes, carrot and peas to the Instant Pot Ace Blender.
2. Pulse until fully combined.
3. Stir in the rest of the ingredients except the cheese.
4. Press soup setting and set it to 15:00 minutes.
5. Top with the cheese and serve.

Serving Suggestions: Garnish with chopped fresh herbs.

Preparation & Cooking Tips: You can also sauté onion and garlic before adding to the blender.

# Red Pepper Soup

Preparation Time: 15 minutes

Cooking Time: 15 minutes

Servings: 4

Ingredients:

- 2 lb. red bell peppers, roasted
- 1 tablespoon vegetable oil
- Garlic salt to taste
- 4 cups vegetable broth

Method:

1. Add red bell peppers and oil to the Instant Pot Ace Blender.
2. Press pulse and then start.
3. Pulse until smooth.
4. Add garlic salt and vegetable broth.
5. Press soup function.
6. Set it to 15:00 minutes.

Serving Suggestions: Garnish with chopped red bell peppers.

Preparation & Cooking Tips: You can also use yellow and green bell peppers for this recipe.

# Broccoli Soup

Preparation Time: 15 minutes

Cooking Time: 15 minutes

Servings: 4

Ingredients:

- 2 tablespoons olive oil
- 4 cups broccoli
- Salt and pepper to taste
- 1 teaspoon thyme dried
- 3 cups water
- 1 cup cream

Method:

1. Add oil and broccoli to the Instant Pot Ace Blender.
2. Press pulse and start.
3. Pulse until fully ground.
4. Stir in the rest of the ingredients.
5. Choose soup setting.
6. Set it to 15:00 minutes.

Serving Suggestions: Sprinkle with fresh thyme leaves on top.

Preparation & Cooking Tips: Use low-fat cream.

# Chapter 4: Dips

## Spinach & Artichoke Dip

Preparation Time: 10 minutes

Cooking Time: 0 minute

Servings: 8

Ingredients:

- 4 oz. cream cheese
- 2 cups plain Greek yogurt
- 1 tablespoon honey
- 1/2 teaspoon Worcestershire sauce
- 1/4 cup Parmesan cheese, grated
- 1 teaspoon onion powder
- Salt and pepper to taste
- 14 oz. canned artichoke hearts, rinsed and drained
- 2 cups spinach

Method:

1. Put all the ingredients except artichoke and spinach to the Instant Pot Ace Blender.
2. Seal the blender.
3. Press pulse.
4. Pulse until smooth.
5. Press pause.
6. Add artichoke and spinach.
7. Pulse until fully combined.

Serving Suggestions: Serve with baked chips or vegetable dippers.

Preparation & Cooking Tips: Chill before serving.

# Marinara Sauce

Preparation Time: 15 minutes

Cooking Time: 20 minutes

Servings: 4

Ingredients:

- 2 tablespoons olive oil
- 1 onion, chopped
- 4 cloves garlic, chopped
- 1 carrot, chopped
- 28 oz. canned tomatoes, liquid undrained
- 3 tablespoons tomato paste
- 3 tablespoons fresh basil, chopped
- 1 tablespoon sugar
- 1 teaspoon dried oregano
- Salt and pepper to taste

Method:

1. Combine all the ingredients in the Instant Pot Ace Blender.
2. Lock the lid in place.
3. Choose soup setting.
4. Set it to 20:00 minutes.
5. After 20 minutes, press pulse for 3 seconds.

Serving Suggestions: Serve with bread or pasta.

Preparation & Cooking Tips: You can also add red pepper flakes to the recipe.

# Roasted Red Pepper Sauce

Preparation Time: 10 minutes

Cooking Time: 10 minutes

Servings: 4

Ingredients:

- 2 tablespoons butter
- 3 stalks, green onion, sliced in half
- 4 oz. cream cheese
- 1 cup half and half
- 1/2 cup Parmesan cheese
- 12 oz. roasted red peppers
- Salt and pepper to taste

Method:

1. Stir all the ingredients in the Instant Pot Ace Blender.
2. Seal the blender.
3. Choose puree 2 setting.

Serving Suggestions: Serve with chips or bread.

Preparation & Cooking Tips: You can also add pinch of cayenne pepper to the mix.

# Garlic Hummus

Preparation Time: 15 minutes

Cooking Time: 0 minute

Servings: 4

Ingredients:

- 1 head garlic, roasted and peeled
- 28 oz. chickpeas, rinsed and drained
- 4 tablespoons tahini
- 1/4 cup lemon juice
- 1/4 cup olive oil
- 1/8 teaspoon cayenne pepper
- 1/2 teaspoon cumin
- Salt to taste

Method:

1. Combine all ingredients to the Instant Pot Ace Blender.
2. Seal the blender.
3. Choose medium manual setting.
4. Blend for 1 minute.
5. Press high manual setting.
6. Blend for 2 minutes.

Serving Suggestions: Serve with pita bread, crackers or chips.

Preparation & Cooking Tips: You can also use plain garlic for this recipe.

# Creamy Italian Dip

Preparation Time: 10 minutes

Cooking Time: 0 minute

Servings: 4

Ingredients:

- 1/2 cup olive oil
- 3 tablespoons mayonnaise
- 1/3 cup sour cream
- 2 tablespoons white wine vinegar
- 2 tablespoons red wine vinegar
- 3 tablespoons Parmesan cheese, grated
- 1 teaspoon Dijon mustard
- 1/2 teaspoon garlic salt
- 2 teaspoons honey
- 1/4 teaspoon onion powder
- 3/4 teaspoon dried basil
- 3/4 teaspoon dried parsley
- 1/8 teaspoon cayenne pepper
- 1/8 teaspoon dried oregano
- Pepper to taste

Method:

1. Mix all the ingredients in the Instant Pot Ace Blender.
2. Lock the lid in place.
3. Choose low manual setting.

4. Blend for 5 seconds.

5. Choose high manual setting.

6. Blend for 10 seconds.

Serving Suggestions: Serve with vegetable dippers.

Preparation & Cooking Tips: Use light mayonnaise.

# Avocado Dip

Preparation Time: 15 minutes

Cooking Time: 0 minute

Servings: 6

Ingredients:

- 2 avocado, sliced into cubes
- 1 tablespoon lime juice
- 1 clove garlic
- Salt and pepper to taste
- 1/2 teaspoon paprika
- 1/2 cup plain Greek yogurt

Method:

1. Add avocado, lime juice, garlic, salt, pepper and paprika to the Instant Pot Ace Blender.
2. Press pulse.
3. Blend until smooth.
4. Stir in yogurt.

Serving Suggestions: Serve with chips or crackers.

Preparation & Cooking Tips: You can also use garlic salt in place of salt.

# Onion Dip

Preparation Time: 10 minutes

Cooking Time: 0 minute

Servings: 4

Ingredients:

- 2 tablespoons olive oil
- 3 cups onion, sliced
- 1 cup plain Greek yogurt
- 1/4 cup water
- 1 teaspoon sugar
- Salt and pepper to taste
- Chopped parsley

Method:

1. Combine all the ingredients to the Instant Pot Ace Blender.
2. Press pulse.
3. Blend until fully combined.

Serving Suggestions: Serve with chips or crackers.

Preparation & Cooking Tips: You can also use flaxseed oil.

# Roasted Red Bell Pepper Dip with Walnuts

Preparation Time: 10 minutes

Cooking Time: 10 minutes

Servings: 6

Ingredients:

- 2 cups bell pepper, roasted
- 2 cups walnuts, roasted
- 1 tablespoon olive oil
- 2 cloves garlic, peeled
- 1 tablespoon honey
- 1 tablespoon lemon juice
- 1 teaspoon paprika
- Salt and pepper to taste

Method:

1. Mix all ingredients in the Instant Pot Ace Blender.
2. Press pulse.
3. Blend until fully combined.

Serving Suggestions: Serve with naan or pita bread.

Preparation & Cooking Tips: You can also use regular walnuts.

# Zucchini Dip

Preparation Time: 10 minutes

Cooking Time: 0 minute

Servings: 4

Ingredients:

- 2 cups zucchini, sliced into cubes
- 1 cup sour cream
- Salt and pepper to taste

Method:

1. Mix all ingredients in the Instant Pot Ace Blender.
2. Press pulse.
3. Pulse until smooth.

Serving Suggestions: Serve with chips or crackers.

Preparation & Cooking Tips: You can also use garlic salt as seasoning for this dip.

# Pumpkin Dip

Preparation Time: 10 minutes

Cooking Time: 0 minute

Servings: 4

Ingredients:

- 1/2 cup brown sugar
- 1 cup cream cheese
- 1/2 cup pumpkin, sliced into cubes and boiled
- 1/2 teaspoon ground cinnamon
- 2 teaspoons maple syrup
- 1 teaspoon water

Method:

1. Put all the ingredients in the Instant Pot Ace Blender.
2. Press medium manual setting.
3. Blend for 3 minutes.

Serving Suggestions: Serve with fruit slices.

Preparation & Cooking Tips: Use low-fat cream cheese.

# Chapter 5: Milks

## Walnut Milk

Preparation Time: 1 hour and 5 minutes

Cooking Time: 0 minute

Servings: 2-4

Ingredients:

- 1 cup walnuts
- Warm water
- 47 oz. water

Method:

1. Soak walnuts in warm water for 1 hour.
2. Drain the water.
3. Add to the Instant Pot Ace Blender along with the water.
4. Select nut / oat milk program.
5. Strain mixture using a mesh strainer.

Serving Suggestions: Serve warm.

Preparation & Cooking Tips: You can store mixture for up to 3 days in the refrigerator.

# Rice Milk

Preparation Time: 5 minutes

Cooking Time: 0 minute

Servings: 4

Ingredients:

- 48 oz. water
- 1/2 teaspoon olive oil
- 1/2 cup white rice

Method:

1. Combine water, oil and rice in the Instant Pot Ace Blender.
2. Seal the blender.
3. Choose rice milk program.
4. Press • for white rice.
5. Filter rice milk through a strainer bag.

Serving Suggestions: Serve with crackers.

Preparation & Cooking Tips: You can refrigerate rice milk for up to 4 days.

# Soy Milk

Preparation Time: 5 minutes

Cooking Time: 0 minute

Servings: 4

Ingredients:

- 3/4 cup soy beans
- 48 oz. water

Method:

1. Add ingredients to the Instant Pot Ace Blender.
2. Secure the lid.
3. Choose soy milk setting.
4. Strain the mixture.

Serving Suggestions: Serve warm.

Preparation & Cooking Tips: Soak soybeans in warm water for 1 hour before blending.

# Oat Milk

Preparation Time: 5 minutes

Cooking Time: 0 minute

Servings: 4

Ingredients:

- Warm water
- 1 cup rolled oats
- 1/2 teaspoon oil

Method:

1. Combine ingredients in the Instant Pot Ace Blender.
2. Lock the lid in place.
3. Choose nut / oat milk program.
4. Filter the milk.

Serving Suggestions: Chill before serving.

Preparation & Cooking Tips: You can also use steel cut oats for this recipe.

# Vanilla Almond Milk

Preparation Time: 1 hour and 5 minutes

Cooking Time: 0 minute

Servings: 4

Ingredients:

- Warm water
- 1 cup almonds
- 48 oz. water
- 2 teaspoons vanilla extract
- 1/3 cup granulated sugar

Method:

1. Soak almonds in warm water for 1 hour.
2. Add almonds and water to the Instant Pot Ace Blender.
3. Press nut / oat milk program.
4. Strain the mixture.
5. Put the strained milk back to the blender.
6. Stir in the rest of the ingredients.
7. Choose low manual setting.
8. Blend for 10 seconds.

Serving Suggestions: Chill before serving.

Preparation & Cooking Tips: You can refrigerate this for up to 4 days.

# Hazelnut Milk

Preparation Time: 5 minutes

Cooking Time: 0 minute

Servings: 4

Ingredients:

- Warm water
- 1 cup hazelnuts
- 48 oz. water

Method:

1. Soak hazelnuts in warm water for 1 hour.
2. Drain the water.
3. Put the hazelnuts to the Instant Pot Ace Blender along with the water.
4. Press nut / oat milk setting.
5. Strain mixture using a filter.

Serving Suggestions: Chill before serving. Serve with cookies.

Preparation & Cooking Tips: You can refrigerate this for up to 4 days.

# Cashew Milk

Preparation Time: 5 minutes

Cooking Time: 0 minute

Servings: 4

Ingredients:

- Warm water
- 1 cup cashews
- 48 oz. water

Method:

1. Pour cashews into a bowl with warm water.
2. Soak for 1 hour.
3. Drain the water.
4. Add these to the Instant Pot Ace Blender along with the remaining water.
5. Choose nut / oat milk setting.
6. Strain mixture using a mesh strainer.

Serving Suggestions: Chill before serving.

Preparation & Cooking Tips: Use plain unsalted cashews for this recipe.

# Sunflower Seed Milk

Preparation Time: 5 minutes

Cooking Time: 0 minute

Servings: 4

Ingredients:

- Warm water
- 1 cup sunflower seeds
- 48 oz. water

Method:

1. Add warm water to a bowl.
2. Soak sunflower seeds for 1 hour.
3. Drain the water.
4. Transfer to the Instant Pot Ace Blender along with the water.
5. Select nut / oat milk program.
6. Strain mixture.

Serving Suggestions: Serve with crackers.

Preparation & Cooking Tips: You can refrigerate this for up to 4 days.

# Almond Milk

Preparation Time: 5 minutes

Cooking Time: 0 minute

Servings: 4

Ingredients:

- Warm water
- 1 cup cashews
- 48 oz. water

Method:

1. Add almonds in a bowl with warm water.
2. Soak for 1 hour.
3. Drain the water.
4. Transfer the almonds to the Instant Pot Ace Blender.
5. Pour in the water.
6. Select nut / oat milk function.
7. Strain almond milk mixture.

Serving Suggestions: Chill before serving.

Preparation & Cooking Tips: You can also use this for no-dairy recipes that require almond milk.

# Pumpkin Seed Milk

Preparation Time: 5 minutes

Cooking Time: 0 minute

Servings: 4

Ingredients:

- Warm water
- 1 cup pumpkin seeds
- 48 oz. water

Method:

1. Soak pumpkin seeds in warm water for 1 hour.
2. Drain the water.
3. Add these to the Instant Pot Ace Blender along with the remaining water.
4. Choose nut / oat milk setting.
5. Strain mixture using a mesh strainer.

Serving Suggestions: Serve with crackers.

Preparation & Cooking Tips: You can refrigerate this for up to 4 days.

# Chapter 6: Pureed Food

## Pureed Squash, Peas & Pear

Preparation Time: 5 minutes

Cooking Time: 5 minutes

Servings: 4

Ingredients:

- 1/2 cup squash, sliced into cubes
- 1/2 cup peas
- 1 cup pears, cored and sliced
- 1/2 cup water

Method:

1. Mix all ingredients to the Instant Pot Ace Blender.
2. Seal the blender.
3. Select puree 2 setting.
4. Process.
5. Let cool before serving.

Serving Suggestions: Sprinkle with salt before serving.

Preparation & Cooking Tips: You can add more water if you want thinner consistency.

# Pureed Strawberry

Preparation Time: 5 minutes

Cooking Time: 5 minutes

Servings: 4

Ingredients:

- 4 cups strawberries
- 2 tablespoons granulated sugar
- 2 tablespoons water

Method:

1. Add all the ingredients to the Instant Pot Ace Blender.
2. Seal the blender.
3. Choose puree 2 setting.
4. Transfer to a bowl and let cool.

Serving Suggestions: You can use this as topping for ice cream, waffle or pancake.

Preparation & Cooking Tips: You can also chop strawberries before blending.

# Pumpkin Puree

Preparation Time: 5 minutes

Cooking Time: 5 minutes

Servings: 2

Ingredients:

- 2 cups pumpkin, sliced into cubes
- 3/4 cup water

Method:

1. Put pumpkin and water to the Instant Pot Ace Blender.
2. Lock the lid in place.
3. Choose puree 2 setting.
4. Transfer to a glass jar with lid and let cool before sealing.

Serving Suggestions: Serve with toasted bread or veggie dippers.

Preparation & Cooking Tips: You can sweeten the pumpkin puree with honey.

# Pureed Carrots

Preparation Time: 5 minutes

Cooking Time: 4 minutes

Servings: 3

Ingredients:

- 2 cups carrots, chopped
- 1 cup water

Method:

1. Add carrots and water to the Instant Pot Ace Blender.
2. Choose puree 2 program.
3. Process.
4. Let cool before serving.

Serving Suggestions: Serve with crackers.

Preparation & Cooking Tips: Season with salt or sweeten with honey.

# Apple & Banana Oats

Preparation Time: 5 minutes

Cooking Time: 3 minutes

Servings: 2

Ingredients:

- 1/3 cup oats
- 2 apples, peeled,cored and sliced
- 1 banana, sliced
- 3/4 cup water

Method:

1. Put all the ingredients to the Instant Pot Ace Blender.
2. Select puree 2 setting.
3. Process and serve.

Serving Suggestions: Serve as breakfast.

Preparation & Cooking Tips: You can also add honey to the recipe if you want to sweeten the puree.

# Chapter 7: Snack/Desserts

## Hazelnut Spread

Preparation Time: 10 minutes

Cooking Time: 10 minutes

Servings: 2

Ingredients:

- 2 cups hazelnuts, roasted
- 1/2 cup almond milk
- 1/3 cup maple syrup
- 1 1/2 tablespoon vanilla extract
- 1/2 teaspoon salt
- 1/4 cup cocoa powder

Method:

1. Put roasted hazelnuts in the Instant Pot Ace Blender.
2. Seal the lid.
3. Press nut butter setting.
4. Press start.
5. Blend for 1 minute.
6. Press pause.
7. Scrape the mixture on the sides of the blender.
8. Press start.
9. Process for 1 minute.
10. Stir in the rest of the ingredients.

11. Press start and process for 1 minute.

Serving Suggestions: Serve with crackers or bread slices.

Preparation & Cooking Tips: Adjust sweetness according to your preference by adding more maple syrup.

# Strawberry Panna Cotta

Preparation Time: 4 hours and5 minutes

Cooking Time: 20 minutes

Servings: 6

Ingredients:

- 1/2 cup sugar
- 1 lb. strawberries, sliced in half
- 2 tablespoons cold water
- 1 1/2 teaspoons plain gelatin
- 1 1/2 cups heavy cream
- 1 teaspoon lemon juice

Method:

1. Combine sugar and strawberries in the blender.
2. Cover the blender.
3. Press pulse and then start.
4. Press soup setting twice to set it to creamy soup.
5. Set time to 12:21 minutes.
6. Transfer mixture to a baking pan.
7. Refrigerate for 4 hours before serving.

Serving Suggestions: Garnish with chopped berries.

Preparation & Cooking Tips: You can also use flavored gelatin to get a tastier panna cotta.

# Pineapple Sorbet

Preparation Time: 10 hours and 15 minutes

Cooking Time: 0 minutes

Servings: 4

Ingredients:

- 3 cups pineapple juice
- 3tablespoons sugar
- 2 tablespoons amaretto liqueur

Method:

1. Mix sugar in pineapple juice and liqueur until the sugar has been dissolved.
2. Pour the mixture into ice cube tray.
3. Freeze for 6 hours.
4. Add frozen ice cubes to blender.
5. Seal the blender.
6. Press crushed ice.
7. Press start.
8. Push ice using the tamper.
9. Repeat until smooth.

Serving Suggestions: Garnish with pineapple slice.

Preparation & Cooking Tips: Use unsweetened pineapple juice.

# Mixed Nut Butter

Preparation Time: 10 minutes

Cooking Time: 10 minutes

Servings: 3

Ingredients:

- 3 cups mixed nuts, roasted
- 3 tablespoon almond oil
- Salt to taste

Method:

1. Put all the ingredients in the Instant Pot Ace Blender.
2. Cover the blender.
3. Blend using medium manual setting.
4. Process for 5 seconds.
5. Press cancel and scrape down on the sides.
6. Repeat several more times until mixture is turned into paste.
7. Process on medium manual setting for 40 seconds.
8. Process on high for 3 minutes.

Serving Suggestions: Serve with crackers or toasted bread.

Preparation & Cooking Tips: You can also use whatever types of nuts you like for making this nut butter.

# Peanut Butter

Preparation Time: 10 minutes

Cooking Time: 10 minutes

Servings: 3

Ingredients:

- 3 cups peanuts, roasted
- 3 tablespoons peanut oil
- Pinch salt

Method:

1. Put all the ingredients in the Instant Pot Ace Blender.
2. Lock the lid in place.
3. Blend using medium manual setting for 5 seconds.
4. Press stop.
5. Scrape the sides.
6. Put the lid back on.
7. Repeat the steps.
8. Blend on medium manual setting for 40 seconds.
9. Choose high and process for 3 minutes.

Serving Suggestions: Serve with banana slices or with toasted bread.

Preparation & Cooking Tips: You can process longer until consistency preferred is reached.

# Conclusion

Blenders have evolved to become great workhorses in the kitchen. Gone are the days when we only whip out the blender to make smoothies.

Now, we even cook soups with it.

The Instant Pot Ace blender is one of the best in making creamy soups, milk alternatives, smoothies, baby food, sauces, and dips.

If you are someone who constantly consumes store-bought milk alternatives, or you just love to eat soup a lot, then the Instant Pot Ace blender is perfect for you. You can make your all-natural milk and velvety smooth soups at the comfort of your own home anytime by just a single push of a button.

Make an oat breakfast bowl in the morning, have smoked sausage chili for lunch, then maybe some chilled late-afternoon margaritas and yummy nachos.

In the evening, make some Manhattan clam chowder and blueberry cheesecake ice cream for dessert. You can make flavorful dishes all-day with this powerful and easy-to-use cooking blender.

CPSIA information can be obtained
at www.ICGtesting.com
Printed in the USA
LVHW061933150122
708507LV00008B/381